Beyond Bilateral Stimulation

Integrating EMDR with Somatic and
Mindfulness Techniques to Heal Trauma
Somatically, Cognitively, and Spiritually for
Whole-Self Transformation

Ray Maritere McLaughlan

The information and resources provided in " Beyond Bilateral Simulation" are for educational and informational purposes only and are not intended as a substitute for professional medical advice, diagnosis, or treatment. The author is not engaged in rendering medical, psychological, or other professional services through this workbook.

The author has taken care to present the information and techniques accurately and responsibly, but they make no representations or warranties of any kind, express or implied, about the completeness, accuracy, reliability, suitability, or availability of the information, products, services, or related graphics contained in the book.

The case studies and examples presented in this book are composite narratives drawn from the author's professional experience, and do not represent any single individual. They are intended for educational purposes only, to illustrate the principles and practices of the Beyond Bilateral approach.

If you have any concerns about your mental health or are experiencing severe or persistent symptoms of anxiety, please consult with a qualified healthcare professional before beginning any self-help program or making changes to your treatment plan

ISBN: 978-1-7640190-6-4

TherapyBooks Publishing

Table of Contents

Preface 1

Chapter 1 Introduction 5

Chapter 2 Foundations 11

Chapter 3 The Beyond Bilateral Methodology 22

Chapter 4 Protocols for Specific Traumas 30

Chapter 5 Mindfulness and Self-Compassion Practices 40

Chapter 6 Resilience and Post-Traumatic Growth 48

Conclusion 59

Reference 65

Preface

Welcome, brave traveler, to the world of healing beyond limits, beyond boundaries, beyond the confines of the ordinary. Welcome to the world of Beyond Bilateral - a world where the power of EMDR meets the wisdom of somatic therapy and the grace of mindfulness, birthing a new paradigm of trauma recovery and personal transformation.

If you've picked up this book, chances are you're no stranger to the ravages of trauma. Maybe you're a survivor yourself, battling the demons of PTSD, anxiety, depression, or chronic pain. Maybe you're a therapist, seeking new ways to help your clients reclaim their lives from the shadow of past wounds. Or maybe you're just a curious soul, drawn to the mysteries of the mind-body connection and the resilience of the human spirit.

Whoever you are, and wherever you find yourself on the journey of healing, know this: you are not alone. You are part of a rising tide of awakening, a global movement of individuals and communities daring to face their darkness, embrace their light, and birth a new way of being in the world.

And that is precisely what this book is about. It's about transcending the limitations of any single modality or approach, and discovering the alchemical magic that happens when we integrate the best of what works. It's about harnessing the power of neuroplasticity, somatic awareness, and mindful presence to rewire our brains, heal our bodies, and liberate our souls. It's about daring to envision a world where wholeness is the norm, not the exception - and then rolling up our sleeves and making it happen, one courageous step at a time.

But let's be real: this journey is not for the faint of heart. Trauma work is deep, raw, and often messy. It requires us to face our deepest fears, feel our most intense emotions, and brave the uncharted territories of our own psyches. It demands that we let go of our familiar patterns and defenses, and open ourselves to new ways of being that may feel foreign, even terrifying at first.

In short, trauma healing is a hero's journey - and like any hero's journey, it comes with its share of trials, tribulations, and dark nights of the soul. But here's the good news: you don't have to walk this path alone. With the right tools, the right support, and the right mindset, you can navigate even the thorniest of terrains with grace, resilience, and even a sense of adventure.

And that's where Beyond Bilateral comes in. Born from the crucible of clinical experience and personal transformation, this approach represents the leading edge of trauma therapy - a synthesis of the most effective, evidence-based practices for healing mind, body, and soul. From the bilateral stimulation of EMDR to the body-based practices of Somatic Experiencing to the compassionate awareness of mindfulness, Beyond Bilateral offers a comprehensive roadmap for the journey of healing - a roadmap that is at once deeply practical and wildly visionary.

But don't just take my word for it. The proof, as they say, is in the pudding - or in this case, in the lives of the countless individuals who have walked this path and emerged on the other side, forever changed. Throughout this book, you'll encounter real-life stories of healing and transformation that will inspire you, challenge you, and remind you of what's possible when we have the courage to face our demons and claim our divinity.

2

You'll also look at the cutting-edge science and theory behind the Beyond Bilateral approach, exploring topics like polyvagal theory, interpersonal neurobiology, and the psychophysiology of trauma. But don't worry - we'll keep things accessible, engaging, and even a bit irreverent. Because let's face it: trauma work is heavy stuff, and a little humor goes a long way in keeping us sane and centered.

Most importantly, you'll walk away from this book with a toolbox full of practical skills and strategies for navigating the ups and downs of trauma recovery. From EMDR protocols to somatic practices to mindfulness meditations, you'll have everything you need to start implementing the Beyond Bilateral approach in your own life or clinical practice right away.

But Beyond Bilateral is more than just a collection of tools and techniques. It's a way of being, a way of relating to ourselves and the world that is rooted in compassion, curiosity, and radical acceptance. It's a path of awakening that invites us to embrace the full spectrum of our humanity - the light and the dark, the beautiful and the broken, the sacred and the profane.

Ultimately, Beyond Bilateral Stimulation is an invitation to come home to ourselves - to reconnect with the deepest truth of who we are, beneath the layers of trauma and conditioning. It's a call to remember our inherent wholeness, our unbreakable resilience, our indestructible essence. And it's a challenge to live from that place of wholeness, to embody our highest potential in service of a world that desperately needs our light.

So if you're ready to take the leap - to go beyond the limits of what you thought was possible and discover a whole new way of being - then welcome, my friend. Welcome to the path of Beyond Bilateral.

May this book be a beacon of hope, a source of guidance, and a companion on the journey. May it illuminate the darkness, ease the suffering, and reveal the brilliance that lies within.

And may you always remember: you are the hero of your own story. You have the power to heal, to thrive, to rise.

The world is waiting for you.

Let's begin.

Ray Maritere McLaughlan

Chapter 1 Introduction

Well, well, well! You've picked up this book, so I assume you're interested in this newfangled "Beyond Bilateral" approach to healing trauma. Good for you! Trauma is a beast that can really mess up your mental and emotional plumbing. But take heart - EMDR (Eye Movement Desensitization and Reprocessing) offers some serious relief. And when you mix in somatic and mindfulness practices, hoo-boy, get ready for a whole new level of healing!

The Juice on EMDR, Somatic Work & Mindfulness

Let me give you the straight dope on why integrating EMDR with body-based and mindful approaches is the cat's pajamas:

EMDR, as you may know, is a well-researched therapy that uses eye movements (or other bilateral stimulation) to reprocess distressing memories. It's like sending your brain to the dry cleaners - those gnarly trauma stains get lifted right out! Clients often feel a big shift in perspective and a lightening of their emotional load. Nifty, right?

But here's the rub: Trauma isn't just in your head. It gets stored in your body too, like gum stuck to the bottom of your shoe. You can't just think your way to freedom - you gotta feel it in your bones! That's where somatic (body-based) methods come in. They help you release all that pent-up survival energy and tension so you can finally relax, for crying out loud!

Mindfulness is the secret sauce that helps you stay cool and collected as you do this deep diving. By paying attention to the present moment (instead of getting hijacked by the past), you can navigate those tricky trauma waters with more ease. It's like having a wise, compassionate friend in your corner, reminding you that you're basically okay, even when the going gets tough.

So when you roll EMDR, somatic work, and mindfulness into one tasty healing burrito, you're covering all your bases - mental, physical, and spiritual. It's a whole-person approach to whooping trauma's butt!

My Own Adventures in Healing La-La Land

Now, I know what you might be thinking: "Easy for you to say, Mr. Smarty-Pants Therapist! What do you know about trauma?" Well, let me tell you, I've earned my badges in the healing trenches. My own noggin has been through the wringer!

You see, I'm a card-carrying member of the Complex PTSD club (childhood trauma division). For years, I hauled around a whole stagecoach of traumatic baggage - anxiety, depression, dissociation, the whole kit and caboodle. I was a hot mess, stumbling through life in a fog of unresolved pain. Talk about a party! (Not).

Well, I finally got fed up with my own tomfoolery and jumped on the therapy bandwagon. I tried all the usual suspects - CBT, talk therapy, support groups. And while they helped me understand my issues (and made for excellent self-help cocktail party banter), I still felt stuck in the muck.

Then I discovered EMDR. Hot dog! Those bi-lateral eye movements were like windshield wipers for my brain - clearing away the trauma residue so I could see my life with fresh peepers. I started to feel more present, grounded, and dare I say, hopeful.

But my body was still doing the post-traumatic polka - tight shoulders, churning guts, the whole shebang. I needed to get out of my head and into my soma! So I added somatic experiencing (SE) to my healing repertoire. Slowly but surely, I learned to track my body's sensations, discharge that old stuck energy, and come home to myself in a whole new way.

Mindfulness tied it all together like a bright red bow. By learning to observe my inner world with curiosity and compassion (instead of judgement and shame), I discovered I could be with my painful bits without drowning in the drama. It was like finding a life raft of peaceful presence amidst the stormy trauma seas.

Lo and behold, this perfect storm of EMDR, SE, and mindfulness practices truly transformed my inner landscape (and made me much better company at dinner parties)! My traumatic memories lost their electric charge, my nervous system settled into a groovy "rest and digest" rhythm, and I felt a sense of wholeness and resilience I'd never known before. Hot diggity!

You Too Can Be a Healing Hero!

Now, I know what you're thinking - "That's swell for you, but what about little ol' me?" Fear not, my friend! The brave new world of Beyond Bilateral healing is available to all who dare to step onto the path.

I've worked with countless clients who've been through the trauma wringer - childhood abuse, sexual assault, war vets, you name it. And time after time, I've seen the magic of integrating EMDR with somatic and mindful practices work its mojo.

Take my client, "Sarah" (not her real name, obviously. I don't fancy getting sued!). Sarah was a walking poster child for complex PTSD - dissociation, hypervigilance, emotional numbness, the full enchilada. She'd been through the therapy gauntlet but still felt haunted by her past.

Well, we started with some good old-fashioned EMDR to clear the cognitive cobwebs. And sure enough, Sarah began to process her traumatic memories with more clarity and less distress. But her body was still bracing for impact, like a soldier in the trenches.

So we added some SE to the mix, guiding Sarah to notice her physical sensations and release the trapped survival energy through gentle shaking and breath. Over time, her system settled and she felt more grounded in her skin.

But the real magic happened when Sarah developed a mindfulness practice. By learning to meet her experience with loving awareness (instead of resistance and rumination), she discovered an unshakeable core of okayness, even in the face of difficult feelings.

Slowly but surely, Sarah learned to re-inhabit her body, mind, and spirit as an integrated whole. Her PTSD symptoms faded into the background, and a profound sense of peace and vitality blossomed. She went from surviving to thriving, one courageous healing step at a time.

And that, my friends, is the promise of Beyond Bilateral work. By weaving together the power of EMDR, somatic approaches, and mindfulness, we can heal trauma at the deepest roots and awaken to our birthright of joyful aliveness. No matter how lost in the underworld of PTSD you may feel, there is a way home to wholeness.

So if you're ready to leave the trauma merry-go-round and step into a brave new world of body-mind-spirit healing, you've come to the right place! This book will be your trusty trail guide, offering a clear, step-by-step path through the dense forest of trauma recovery. Along the way, we'll explore:

- The nuts and bolts of EMDR, somatic work, and mindfulness - what they are, how they work, and why they're a match made in heaven

- Practical tools and practices you can use right away to start feeling better in your skin and your psyche

- Real-life case studies (with the names changed to protect the innocent!) to illustrate the healing process in action

- Common pitfalls and how to navigate them with grit and grace

- How to find the right support team to champion your healing journey

- And so much more!

I won't lie - the terrain of trauma healing is no walk in the park. It takes guts, gumption, and a whole lotta patience. But if you're willing to roll up your sleeves, face your demons with courage and compassion, and stay the course, the rewards are beyond measure. You can reclaim your birthright of wholeness, vitality, and unshakeable resilience. You can finally come home to yourself, in all your glorious imperfection.

And really, what could be more worthwhile than that?

So grab a beverage, find a cozy spot, and let's sally forth into the wild and wonderful world of Beyond Bilateral healing. Your brave new life awaits!

Conclusion

Healing trauma is not for the faint of heart. It requires a willingness to face the pain of the past, to feel it fully, and to release it layer by layer. EMDR, somatic work, and mindfulness are powerful allies in this process, offering a clear path out of post-traumatic purgatory.

By integrating these modalities, we have the opportunity to rewire our minds, bodies, and spirits for wholeness and resilience. We can move from surviving to thriving, from post-traumatic stress to post-traumatic growth.

No matter how far down the rabbit hole of trauma you may have fallen, this book is here to remind you that there is always a way back to the light. With courage, compassion, and the right tools, you can heal at the deepest levels and reclaim your birthright of joyful aliveness.

So here's to the journey ahead - to facing our demons, embracing our wholeness, and daring to live and love with a wide-open heart. The adventure of a lifetime awaits!

Chapter 2 Foundations

Let's establish the essential knowledge you need to understand and apply the Beyond Bilateral approach effectively. We'll cover the basics of EMDR, the crucial mind-body connection in trauma, introductions to somatic experiencing and mindfulness, and key neuroscience principles. With these foundations, you'll have a solid framework for integrating EMDR with somatic and mindful practices.

Overview of EMDR Therapy and Bilateral Stimulation

EMDR (Eye Movement Desensitization and Reprocessing) is an evidence-based therapy for resolving symptoms of traumatic stress and other psychological conditions. Developed by Francine Shapiro, EMDR uses bilateral stimulation, usually side-to-side eye movements, while the client focuses on a disturbing memory. This combination of attention to the memory and bilateral stimulation enables the brain to reprocess the memory, releasing distress and instilling adaptive beliefs.

The key steps in EMDR include:

1. Client history and treatment planning

2. Preparation to establish safety and stabilization skills

3. Assessment to activate the target memory and identify related beliefs

4. Desensitization with bilateral stimulation to reprocess the memory

5. Installation to strengthen positive beliefs

6. Body scan to clear any residual disturbance

7. Closure to ensure equilibrium and between-session resources

8. Re-evaluation at the next session

EMDR's efficacy comes from how it harnesses the brain's natural healing processes. The bilateral stimulation, whether eye movements, taps or tones, creates an alternating activation of the right and left hemispheres. This accelerates memory processing by calling up associated material, forging new neural connections, and integrating the memories into semantic networks.

Research indicates EMDR leads to rapid decreases in subjective distress, reduces trauma symptoms like flashbacks and nightmares, and changes negative beliefs. Clients often report feeling "unstuck" from painful past experiences. While EMDR doesn't erase memories, it defuses their emotional charge so they become less disruptive.

However, EMDR's focus on mental reprocessing doesn't always address how trauma is stored in the body. For a more complete resolution, we need to widen our lens to the somatic dimensions of healing.

The Mind-Body Connection in Trauma and Emotional Healing

Here's the simple truth: You can't separate the mind from the body when it comes to trauma. Traumatic events impact us on multiple levels - mental, emotional, physical and even spiritual. When we go through something horrific or overwhelming, it doesn't just distress our thoughts and feelings. It also leaves imprints in our bodies and nervous systems that shape how we function long after the threat has passed.

Take the story of my client Sarah. Sarah grew up with a violent, alcoholic father who would fly into rages and beat her and her siblings. Even though she's now a successful adult in a safe environment, Sarah's body still carries the residue of those early experiences. She has chronic tension in her shoulders, a tight belly, and shallow breathing. Her nervous system stays on high alert, reacting to small stresses as if they were life-or-death threats.

Sarah's mind understands she's no longer in danger. She's done plenty of good cognitive work to challenge her distorted beliefs and learn healthy coping skills. But her body hasn't gotten the message. It's still armored in a defensive freeze response, bracing against attack. This somatic memory of the trauma keeps her stuck in cycles of anxiety, mistrust and depletion despite her rational understanding.

This is a perfect example of how trauma lives not just in our minds, but in the very cells of our bodies. When we go through something terrifying or overwhelming, our threat detection system gets flipped on and our nervous system mobilizes to protect us. Stress hormones like cortisol and adrenaline flood our body to give us the energy to fight or flee.

If we can't complete that survival response and discharge the energy, it stays stuck in our body. Our muscles stay tense and braced for action. Our digestion shuts down to conserve resources. We dissociate from bodily sensations to block out pain. The traumatic activation gets woven into our posture, breathing, and instinctive reactions. It becomes the new normal.

So we can talk through the traumatic memories and learn to reframe our thoughts, but until we address the somatic roots, full healing remains elusive. The body will continue to sound the trauma alarm and shape our lived experience, often outside cognitive awareness.

This is why EMDR, while powerful, has its limits. The bilateral stimulation can help reprocess traumatic material and update negative beliefs at the mind level. But it doesn't necessarily reach into the trauma capsules stored in the body. We need body-based tools to fully renegotiate and release those deeper contractions.

Enter somatic psychology and mindfulness as crucial allies in whole-person trauma healing. By extending our awareness and intervention to the body and nervous system, we can illuminate and untangle the physical knots of trauma. We open new possibilities for present-moment wholeness and ease that transcend the painful past. So let's explore how these approaches complement EMDR beautifully to connect the dots between mind and body in emotional healing.

Introduction to Somatic Experiencing and Mindfulness

Somatic Experiencing is a pioneering body-based therapy for healing trauma developed by Peter Levine. It starts from this core insight: Trauma is not just a mental event, but a full-body experience that requires a somatic resolution. Mental processing alone can't reach and unwind the instinctive defenses held in the body.

Somatic Experiencing (SE) teaches us to track sensation, witness the body's stress responses, and support the nervous system to complete survival energies in a safe way. Through guided mindfulness, micro-movements, breathwork, and self-touch, SE helps the body release trauma-bound tension and regain its inherent capacity for regulation and aliveness.

Here are the key principles of SE:

1. **Titration**: Moving slowly, in small increments, to avoid overwhelming the nervous system as it touches into distressing activation. Building tolerance bit by bit.

2. **Pendulation**: Guiding attention rhythmically between resources and distress, expansion and contraction, to widen the capacity to stay present and regulated.

3. **Resourcing**: Connecting to positive or neutral sensations, people, places or experiences to counterbalance traumatic activation and build stability.

4. **Discharge**: Allowing the body to complete motor responses of fight/flight/freeze to let go of stuck survival energy through shaking, trembling, heat, tingling.

5. **Settling**: Tracking the body's return to balance as the nervous system unwinds, often marked by deeper breaths, relaxation, a sense of flow.

A skilled SE practitioner acts as a witness and guide, listening to the body's cues and supporting it to renegotiate trauma in its own organic way. There's an honouring of the wisdom of the organism to heal given the right conditions and pacing.

Here's how it worked for my client Sarah:

As Sarah learned to track her body's sensations and stress reactions mindfully, she started noticing the chronic tension she carried from her childhood trauma. When she tuned into her tight shoulders, she felt an urge to punch and push away - the fight response her body never got to complete with her abusive father.

With my guidance, Sarah made small pushing motions with her arms, staying connected to sensation and breath. She experienced trembling, shaking and eventually a flooding of heat as her body discharged the pent-up survival energy. In the settling afterwards, she felt a new spaciousness and ease like a weight had been lifted. Her shoulders softened, her chest opened, her belly relaxed.

This vignette demonstrates SE's power to pick up where talk leaves off. By contacting the somatic residue of trauma and allowing it to release in present time, Sarah experienced a palpable shift that language alone couldn't reach. Her mind-body reunited in a felt sense of relief and wholeness.

So how do we bring this body wisdom to potentize EMDR? By weaving SE skills into all phases, but especially:

- During preparation, to build somatic awareness and regulation capacity
- When distress arises in desensitization, to titrate and discharge activation
- In installation, to fully embody positive cognition in posture and breath
- At closure, to guide the body back to balance through resourcing
- Between sessions, as homework to deepen mind-body integration

Leveraging SE expands EMDR's reach beyond mental reprocessing to the often-overlooked domain of the body. It grounds the shifts in sensate, here-and-now experience. The synergy of EMDR and SE forges the golden link between implicit and explicit memory, left and right brain, thoughts and felt sense in trauma resolution.

Just as EMDR and SE are natural allies, mindfulness beautifully complements them both as a foundational practice for whole-person healing. At its essence, mindfulness simply means paying attention to the present moment with openness and curiosity. By cultivating this non-judgmental quality of attention, we contact reality as it is, beyond the filters of past conditioning.

With trauma, mindful awareness builds our capacity to:

- Notice body sensations, emotions, and thoughts with friendly interest

- Dis-identify from the trauma story and contact a deeper sense of presence

- Bring compassion to wounded parts while accessing inner resources

- Regulate the nervous system through the power of grounded attention

- Reconnect with the body as an ally and messenger of wholeness

Ultimately, mindfulness is a way of coming home to ourselves and discovering that even in the midst of pain, there is an unbroken dimension of basic okayness. We are not defined by our traumas and defenses. They are waves arising in the larger ocean of our being that can be witnessed and held with kindness.

Anchoring EMDR in mindful awareness, we approach the traumatic material from this spacious "witness" consciousness. We're able to be with the activation without drowning in it, and access healing resources at the core. Mindfulness gives us the steadiness to do the difficult work of trauma processing while recognizing our true identity beyond the traumatized self.

So in the Beyond Bilateral approach, we include practices like:

- Mindful tracking of sensations during bilateral stimulation

- Breath-focused meditation to prepare the nervous system

- Compassionate dialogue with activated inner parts

- Body scans to cultivate embodied presence

- Heartfelt resourcing with positive qualities and memories

Folding mindfulness into EMDR in these ways, we help clients contact their innate regulation and resilience. We open portals to the lucidity and love beneath the traumatic debris. This is the foundation for deep, abiding healing that sticks.

Putting It All Together: Rewiring the Traumatized Brain

On the topic of "sticking," let's look at the final puzzle piece of our Beyond Bilateral foundations: Harnessing neuroplasticity to install whole-person healing in the brain and being.

Here's the great news from neuroscience: The brain is changeable. It's constantly laying down new neural pathways based on what we give attention to. This means the patterns of traumatic activation, while deeply grooved, are not fixed. With the right interventions, we can rewire those ruts and encode new possibilities.

EMDR's bilateral stimulation capitalizes on this neuroplasticity by calling up adaptive information and forging associative links in memory networks. The traumatic material gets metabolized and assimilated into a new gestalt.

Adding SE amplifies this rewiring by bringing the body along for the ride. By mindfully contacting somatic activation and "completing the cycle," we lay down fresh imprints of safety, connection and mastery. We move from a trauma-bound state to the lively flow of resilience.

Then with mindfulness, we strengthen the neural circuits of present-moment, compassionate awareness. We encode a sense of self and reality beyond traumatic identity, like overlaying a new program onto a glitchy hard drive.

The big "aha" here is that mind, body, and brain are an interconnected loop. By intervening skillfully at any point on the loop, we affect the whole system. EMDR lights up the mental networks, SE addresses the physiology, and mindfulness brings in the regulating power of attention. Together, they synergize to reboot the entire organism.

It's like we're sending the message to every cell and synapse that the trauma is over, and we can update our operating system to current reality. The beyond bilateral approach surrounds the trauma and its somatic roots with resources for healing, and integrates them into a new narrative and felt sense.

Little by little, this comprehensive rewiring moves traumatic memory into the rearview and awakens innate wholeness in the foreground. Clients shift from living in traumatic trance to embodying their authentic range of aliveness. It's a profound reclamation of self and sovereignty.

This is the vision and promise of EMDR integrated with somatic and mindful approaches. By engaging the natural plasticity of mind and body, we midwife whole-being breakthroughs and a return to intrinsic okayness. It takes dedicated practice, but step by step, the path leads to freedom.

Key Takeaways

So, friends, let's review the key foundations of our Beyond Bilateral paradigm:

1. EMDR uses bilateral stimulation to reprocess traumatic memories and encode adaptive information, harnessing the brain's innate healing capacities.

2. Trauma is stored not just in the mind, but in the body's nervous system and implicit memories. Somatic approaches like Somatic Experiencing access and renegotiate this physiological activation for fuller resolution.

3. Mindfulness builds the capacity to witness trauma and contact healing presence. It is the essential ground for whole-person healing.

4. The brain is changeable. EMDR, SE and mindfulness work together to rewire neural networks and shift the operating system from trauma to resilience.

5. Integrating EMDR with somatic and mindful tools creates a powerful synergy that reaches the mental, physical and spiritual dimensions of trauma for deep, lasting transformation.

Take heart! While trauma and the path to healing can feel overwhelming at times, these insights and practices are your trusty allies. By exploring this terrain with courage and compassion, you move ever closer to the intrinsic ease, aliveness and wholeness of your true nature.

So let's roll up our sleeves and look at how to actually apply these principles in the transformative journey of Beyond Bilateral healing. Onward!

Chapter 3 The Beyond Bilateral Stimulation Methodology

Alrighty then! Now that we've laid the conceptual groundwork, it's time to roll up our sleeves and get down to the nitty-gritty of how to actually do this Beyond Bilateral Stimulation mojo. In this chapter, we'll examine the core techniques and protocols, how to artfully merge together EMDR with somatic and mindfulness practices, and some juicy case studies to bring it all to life. So put on your thinking caps and let's get cracking!

The Beyond Bilateral Stimulation Tango: A Step-by-Step Guide

First things first: The foundation of the Beyond Bilateral approach is good old-fashioned EMDR. If you're not already trained in EMDR, stop right there! Go get trained by a reputable organization and come back when you've got that under your belt. We'll wait.

Okay, now that we've got that out of the way, here's the basic steps of the Beyond Bilateral shuffle:

1. **Phase 1: History Taking.** You know the drill - gather info about your client's presenting issues, trauma history, and current functioning. But don't just focus on the facts, ma'am! Tune into their body language, emotional tenor, and any signs of dissociation. This will give you clues about where to focus your somatic and mindfulness interventions down the line.

2. **Phase 2: Preparation.** Here's where we start weaving in the somatic and mindful elements. Teach your client some basic grounding and centering techniques (more on that in a bit). Help them cultivate a friendly

relationship with their body and breath. This will create a solid foundation of safety and stabilization.

3. **Phase 3: Assessment.** Identify the target memory, the neggy coggy (that's psychobabble for negative cognition), and the desired positive belief. But don't stop there! Check in with the body. Where do they feel the distress? What sensations arise? This will give you a roadmap for where to direct the somatic work.

4. **Phase 4: Desensitization.** Ah, the meat and potatoes of EMDR! Guide your client to focus on the target memory while doing the ol' bilateral stimulation (eye movements, taps, or tones). But here's the twist: Encourage them to notice any body sensations that arise, without judgment. If they start to feel overwhelmed, take a break and do some somatic resourcing (again, more on that soon).

5. **Phase 5: Installation.** Once the distress is down to a 0 or 1 (on that trusty 0-10 SUDs scale), it's time to install the positive belief. But don't just have them repeat it like a parrot! Encourage them to really feel it in their body. Where do they sense the truth of that statement? How does it land somatically? This will help anchor the new belief on a visceral level.

6. **Phase 6: Body Scan.** This is where the magic happens! Guide your client to scan their body from head to toe, noticing any residual tension, tightness, or other sensations. If they find a spot that still holds some charge, do some focused somatic release work (yup, you guessed it - more deets coming up!).

7. **Phase 7: Closure.** Make sure your client is grounded and centered before they leave your office. Do a final mind-body check-in. Give them some resources to take home (a relaxation audio, a grounding exercise, a mindfulness app recommendation). Remind them that processing continues between sessions, so be extra kind to themselves.

8. **Phase 8: Re-evaluation.** Check in at the beginning of the next session. How did they fare in the real world? Any new insights, body shifts, or emotional releases? Use this intel to guide your next round of Beyond Bilateral work.

Rinse and repeat, my friends! With each cycle of this process, the trauma networks get desensitized, the positive beliefs get installed, and the body-mind returns to a more regulated, resilient state. It's a beautiful thing to behold.

Mixing It Up: Blending EMDR with Somatic and Mindful Mojo

Now, you might be wondering: "How exactly do I incorporate somatic and mindfulness techniques into this process? Do I just throw them in willy-nilly?" Fear not, dear reader - there's a method to the madness!

Here are some key ways to seamlessly integrate body-based and mindful practices into your EMDR work:

- **Grounding and Centering.** Teach your clients simple techniques to land in the here-and-now, like feeling their feet on the ground, noticing their breath, or doing a quick body scan. Have them practice these regularly, so they become second nature. This will help them stay present and resourced during the EMDR work.

- **Somatic Resourcing.** Help your clients identify positive or neutral sensations in their body (e.g., a sense of warmth in their belly, a tingly aliveness in their hands, a spaciousness in their chest). Encourage them to linger there, really savoring the goodness. This will build their capacity to tolerate distress and rewire their nervous system for safety and ease.

- **Pendulation.** During the desensitization phase, guide your clients to gently shift their attention back and forth between the traumatic material and a resourced state in their body. This "pendulation" helps the system discharge the activation and restore equilibrium. It's like a neural seesaw!

- **Titration.** If your client starts to feel overwhelmed, slow things down. Encourage them to take smaller "bites" of the traumatic memory, while staying anchored in the present moment. This "titration" prevents re-traumatization and allows the processing to unfold at a manageable pace.

- **Mindful Noticing.** Throughout the EMDR process, invite your clients to simply observe their internal experience with curiosity and non-judgment. Encourage them to let the body sensations, images, emotions, and thoughts arise and pass, like waves on the ocean. This mindful stance helps them dis-identify from the trauma and access their innate healing wisdom.

- **Embodied Installation.** When it comes time to install the positive cognition, don't just focus on the words. Guide your clients to feel the resonance of the statement in their body. Where do they sense the truth of it? How does it vibrate in their bones? This somatic anchoring helps the belief "stick" on a deeper level.

- **Compassionate Self-Touch.** If your client is feeling raw or vulnerable after a session, encourage them to place a hand on their heart, belly, or any other soothing spot. This simple act of self-kindness can work wonders to calm the nervous system and promote feelings of safety and connection.

Of course, this is just a sampling of the many ways you can blend EMDR with somatic and mindfulness practices. The key is to get creative, trust your intuition, and adjust based on your client's unique needs and responses. It's more art than science!

Tales from the Trenches: Case Studies of Integration in Action

Enough theory, let's make this real! Here are a couple case vignettes to illustrate how this Beyond Bilateral stuff looks in practice:

Case 1: Sally and the Somatic Shakedown

Sally was a 35-year-old survivor of childhood sexual abuse. She had been in talk therapy for years, but still struggled with debilitating flashbacks, nightmares, and a pervasive sense of shame. When she first came to see me, her body was a bundle of nerves - tight, jittery, and disconnected.

We started with some basic EMDR to process the most distressing memories. Sally courageously faced the abuse experiences, letting the bilateral stimulation work its desensitizing magic. But after a few sessions, we hit a wall. She felt stuck, like the memories were processed but the shame lingered.

That's when we shifted into somatic gear. I guided Sally to notice where she felt the shame in her body - a dense, leaden sensation in her belly. We stayed with that, breathing into it, letting it soften and unfurl. To her amazement, the shame started to dissolve, replaced by a warm tingle of aliveness.

As we continued the EMDR-somatic dance, Sally began to feel more at home in her skin. She even started to experience glimmers of self-love and acceptance - foreign terrain for someone with her trauma history. By the end of our work, she was standing tall, radiating a quiet confidence and ease. Her shame had melted away, and in its place was a deep knowing of her inherent worth.

Case 2: Bob and the Mindful Breakthrough

Bob was a Vietnam vet with a classic case of PTSD - hypervigilance, explosive anger, emotional numbness, the whole shebang. He had tried every treatment under the sun, but nothing seemed to touch the raw nerve of his war trauma.

In our first EMDR session, we homed in on a particularly harrowing firefight memory. As Bob focused on the image, his body started to shake and sweat. His breath became rapid and shallow. He was clearly in the throes of a flashback.

Rather than forging ahead, we took a mindful pause. I guided Bob to feel his feet on the ground, to notice his breath moving in and out. Gradually, his system settled and he was able to return to the present moment.

With this newfound mindful anchor, we gently re-engaged the memory. This time, Bob was able to process it without getting hijacked by the terror. He even started to make meaning of the experience, seeing how it had shaped his identity as a survivor.

As we integrated mindfulness into the EMDR protocol, Bob's capacity to be with his traumatic past expanded exponentially. He learned to observe his triggers with curiosity rather than reactivity. He discovered an inner stillness that could weather any storm.

By the end of our work, Bob was a changed man. He was more relaxed, more connected, more at peace. The war still lived inside him, but it no longer ran the show. With the skillful application of EMDR and mindfulness, he had reclaimed his life and his humanity.

These cases illustrate the power of integrating EMDR with somatic and mindfulness-based practices. By engaging the body and cultivating present-moment awareness, we can catalyze breakthroughs that go beyond mere symptom reduction. We can help our clients heal at the deepest levels, restoring a sense of wholeness and vitality that many trauma survivors have never known.

Bringing It Home

Alright, folks, we've covered a lot of ground in this chapter! We've explored the nitty-gritty of how to integrate EMDR with somatic and mindfulness practices, and we've seen some real-life examples of how this approach can work wonders.

But here's the thing: This Beyond Bilateral stuff isn't a one-size-fits-all protocol. It's a framework, a set of principles and practices that you can adapt to your own unique style and clientele. The key is to stay curious, creative, and attuned to the wisdom of the body-mind.

So as you embark on this Beyond Bilateral journey, remember: Trust the process, trust your instincts, and above all, trust the innate healing capacity of your clients. With a little skill, a lot of heart, and a healthy dose of humility, you can guide them home to their essential wholeness.

And what could be more rewarding than that?

So go forth, brave clinician, and make some Beyond Bilateral magic! Your clients (and their nervous systems) will thank you.

Chapter 4 Protocols for Specific Traumas

Alright, buckle up folks! We've covered the basics of the Beyond Bilateral approach, but now it's time to get specific. Because let's face it - not all traumas are created equal. Childhood abuse, attachment wounds, anxiety disorders - each of these buggers has its own special flavor of awful. So in this chapter, we're going to explore some targeted protocols for these common trauma types. Get ready to take your Beyond Bilateral skills to the next level!

Healing the Wounds of Childhood: Abuse and Neglect

First up, let's talk about the elephant in the room - childhood trauma. Whether it's physical abuse, sexual abuse, emotional abuse, or neglect, these early experiences can leave some seriously deep scars. Scars that can last a lifetime if not properly addressed.

So how do we use the Beyond Bilateral approach to heal these wounds? Here are some key techniques:

1. **Establish Safety.** First and foremost, we need to create a safe, stable, nurturing environment for our clients. Many childhood trauma survivors never had a secure base, so it's our job to provide that. This means going slow, building trust, and being a consistent, reliable presence.

2. **Resource the Child Self.** In EMDR terms, we want to "install" positive resources for the wounded child self. This could be imagining a nurturing adult presence, a safe place, or a protective figure. We can use somatic resourcing to help the client feel these resources in their body.

3. **Process the Trauma.** Once we have a solid foundation of safety and resourcing, we can start to process the traumatic memories. This is where the standard EMDR protocol comes in - desensitizing the memories and installing positive cognitions. But with childhood trauma, we may need to go slower and titrate the processing more.

4. **Integrate the Child Self.** As we process the memories, we also want to help integrate the wounded child self with the adult self. This means acknowledging the pain, validating the emotions, and offering compassion. Somatic techniques like imaginal nurturing touch or dialoguing with the child self can be powerful here.

5. **Strengthen the Adult Self.** Finally, we want to reinforce the client's adult resources and coping skills. This could involve practical strategies like boundary setting, self-care, and assertiveness training. The goal is to help the client feel empowered and equipped to handle life's challenges.

Here's an example of how this might look in practice:

Jenna, a 30-year-old survivor of childhood sexual abuse, came to therapy struggling with depression, anxiety, and intimacy issues. In our early sessions, we focused on building trust and safety. I taught Jenna some grounding techniques and we developed a "safe place" resource - a cozy treehouse where she could feel protected and nurtured.

As we moved into processing the abuse memories, Jenna used the treehouse imagery to titrate the distress. Whenever the processing got too intense, she could visualize climbing up into her treehouse and feeling the warm, supportive presence of her "wise woman" self.

In between sets of bilateral stimulation, we used somatic resourcing to help Jenna feel more stable in her body. She placed her hand on her heart and imagined golden light filling her chest, soothing the frightened child within.

Over time, Jenna was able to fully process the abuse memories and install positive beliefs like "I am safe now" and "I am worthy of love." We also did some inner child work, with Jenna imagining her adult self comforting and protecting her younger self.

By the end of our work together, Jenna reported feeling more grounded, self-assured, and able to set healthy boundaries in her relationships. She no longer felt haunted by her past, but instead felt a sense of pride in her resilience and strength.

Healing childhood wounds is rarely quick or easy, but with the right approach, it is possible. The Beyond Bilateral framework gives us a roadmap for navigating this complex terrain with skill, compassion, and a whole lot of hope.

Mending Broken Bonds: Attachment Trauma and Relational Wounds

Next up, let's explore another common source of trauma - attachment wounds and relational injuries. As human beings, we are wired for connection. We need secure, nurturing bonds to thrive. But what happens when those bonds are broken, either through early childhood experiences or later relational traumas like intimate partner violence or betrayal? The result can be a pervasive sense of disconnection, mistrust, and emotional pain.

So how can we use the Beyond Bilateral approach to mend these broken bonds? Here are some key strategies:

1. **Focus on the Relationship.** With attachment trauma, the relationship itself is often the "target memory." Rather than processing specific incidents, we may need to work with the overall felt sense of the relationship. This means attuning to the client's attachment style and relational needs.

2. **Strengthen the Therapeutic Alliance.** The therapy relationship can be a powerful corrective experience for attachment wounds. By being a consistent, attuned, and empathetic presence, we can help the client internalize a new model of healthy relating. This secure base in the therapy room can then generalize to other relationships.

3. **Use Somatic Interventions.** Attachment trauma lives in the body - in the visceral sensations of longing, fear, shame, and isolation. Somatic techniques can help regulate these overwhelming feelings and restore a sense of safety and connection. This could involve breathwork, body scans, or even safe physical touch (with clear boundaries and consent, of course!).

4. **Practice Relational Mindfulness.** Mindfulness isn't just an individual practice - it can also be a powerful relational tool. By guiding the client to tune into their present-moment experience during interactions (either in the therapy dyad or in their outside relationships), we can help them notice and shift their relational patterns. This could involve tracking bodily sensations, emotions, and impulses in real-time.

5. **Identify and Install Earned Secure Attachment.** Even if a client didn't have a secure attachment in childhood, they can still develop what's known as "earned security" through later corrective experiences. Our job is to help them identify and strengthen these experiences of healthy relating, both in therapy and in their current relationships. We can use EMDR to install positive cognitions around deserving love, being capable of intimacy, and trusting others.

Here's a case example to illustrate these principles in action:

Mark, a 45-year-old man, sought therapy after his wife of 20 years left him for another man. He was devastated by the betrayal and found himself spiraling into a deep depression. As we explored his history, it became clear that Mark had a long-standing pattern of codependent relationships rooted in early attachment wounds.

In our sessions, I focused first on providing a safe, supportive relationship for Mark to grieve the loss of his marriage. I validated his pain and helped him regulate his intense emotions through somatic techniques like deep breathing and progressive muscle relaxation.

As Mark began to stabilize, we started to process his attachment history using EMDR. Rather than focusing on specific memories, we worked with the overall felt sense of insecurity and unworthiness that permeated his relationships. During bilateral stimulation, I guided Mark to notice the sensations in his body and to imagine a nurturing presence coming to comfort his younger self.

In between sessions, I gave Mark homework to practice relational mindfulness. He started to notice his impulses to people-please or to withdraw in his interactions, and to experiment with new, more assertive responses.

Over time, Mark began to develop a stronger sense of self and a more secure attachment style. He started dating again and found himself attracted to healthier partners who respected his boundaries. In our final sessions, we installed positive cognitions like "I am worthy of love" and "I can be myself in relationships."

By the end of therapy, Mark reported feeling more confident, self-assured, and able to navigate the ups and downs of intimacy. He no longer felt defined by his attachment wounds, but instead felt a sense of hard-won security and resilience.

Healing attachment trauma is a gradual process that requires patience, attunement, and a deep respect for the client's relational history. By blending EMDR with somatic and relational techniques, we can help clients rewire their attachment patterns and find the healthy, nurturing connections they deserve.

Taming the Beasts Within: Anxiety, Phobias, Addictions, and Compulsions

Last but not least, let's talk about those pesky internal demons - anxiety, phobias, addictions, and compulsive behaviors. These issues may not be "traumas" in the classic sense, but they can certainly stem from traumatic experiences and cause a whole lot of suffering. And let's be real - who among us hasn't wrestled with one (or more!) of these beasts at some point in our lives?

So how can the Beyond Bilateral approach help tame these unruly critters? Here are some key tactics:

1. **Identify the Root Causes.** Often, anxiety, phobias, addictions, and compulsions are just the tip of the iceberg - the visible symptoms of deeper emotional wounds. Our job is to help the client connect the dots between their current struggles and their past experiences. This could involve exploring family history, attachment patterns, or specific traumatic events.

2. **Desensitize the Triggers.** Using EMDR, we can target and reprocess the specific memories, images, or sensations that trigger the problematic responses. This could be a past humiliation that fuels social anxiety, a childhood accident that sparks a phobia, or a traumatic loss that drives addiction. By desensitizing these triggers, we can help the client break free from their grip.

3. **Install Adaptive Coping Skills.** As we process the underlying traumas, we also want to equip the client with healthier ways of coping with stress and discomfort. This is where cognitive-behavioral techniques come in handy - things like relaxation training, exposure therapy, and thought challenging. We can use EMDR to install these skills as positive resources.

4. **Strengthen Somatic Awareness.** Anxiety, phobias, addictions, and compulsions all have strong physiological components - racing heartbeat, shaky hands, cravings, muscle tension. By teaching the client to tune into their body's signals with curiosity and compassion, we can help them intervene earlier in the cycle. Somatic techniques like body scans, sensory grounding, and breathwork can be game-changers here.

5. **Cultivate Mindful Acceptance.** Ultimately, the goal is not to eliminate all anxiety, fear, or discomfort (that's

impossible!), but rather to change the client's relationship to these experiences. Mindfulness practices can help foster a sense of spacious, non-judgmental awareness that allows room for the full range of human emotions. By learning to coexist with their internal beasts, clients can paradoxically tame them and find greater freedom.

Here's an example of how these principles might look in practice:

Sarah, a 25-year-old grad student, came to therapy seeking help for a debilitating fear of flying. She had been avoiding planes for years, but her anxiety was starting to interfere with her career aspirations and personal life.

As we explored Sarah's history, we uncovered a specific traumatic memory of a turbulent flight she had taken as a child. Sarah vividly remembered the shaking of the plane, the panicked screams of the passengers, and her own sense of sheer terror. This memory had generalized into a pervasive phobia of flying.

Using EMDR, we targeted and reprocessed this specific memory. Sarah courageously allowed herself to re-experience the sensations of that frightening flight, while I guided her to notice her body's responses and to ground herself in the present moment. Gradually, the charge around the memory began to dissipate.

In between sessions, Sarah practiced relaxation techniques and visualized successful flights. We used EMDR to install these positive resources, helping Sarah access a sense of calm and confidence in the face of her fear.

As Sarah's phobia began to lift, we also explored the deeper emotional roots of her anxiety - a history of family instability and a core belief that the world was unsafe. Through a combination of talk therapy, somatic awareness, and mindfulness practices, Sarah started to challenge these old narratives and cultivate a greater sense of inner safety.

By the end of our work together, Sarah was able to take a short flight to visit her sister. She reported feeling anxious, but not overwhelmed. She was able to use her skills to stay grounded and present, even amidst the discomfort. Most importantly, she felt a newfound sense of pride and empowerment in facing her fear head-on.

Overcoming anxiety, phobias, addictions, and compulsions is rarely a linear process. It requires a willingness to confront the things we most want to avoid, and to learn to relate to our internal experiences in a new way. The Beyond Bilateral approach gives us a toolkit for this brave work - a way to process the past, rewire the brain, and cultivate a more peaceful present.

Wrapping It Up

Whew, that was a whirlwind tour of some of the most common and challenging trauma presentations we face as therapists! We covered a lot of ground - childhood abuse, attachment wounds, anxiety, phobias, addictions, and compulsions. And through it all, we saw how the Beyond Bilateral approach can be adapted and applied to meet the unique needs of each client and situation.

The beauty of this approach is its flexibility and integrative nature. By blending the power of EMDR with the wisdom of somatic and mindfulness practices, we have a truly holistic way of healing trauma - one that addresses the mind, body, and spirit.

But let's be real - this work is not for the faint of heart. It requires a willingness to sit with intense emotions, to attune to the body's signals, and to hold space for the client's pain. It demands that we bring our full selves to the therapy room - our knowledge, our skills, and our own hard-won wisdom.

And yet, there is no greater privilege than walking alongside someone on their journey of healing. To witness a client reclaiming their life from the grip of trauma, to see them discover their own inner resources and resilience - it's nothing short of miraculous.

Chapter 5 Mindfulness and Self-Compassion Practices

Alright folks, we've talked a lot about the fancy techniques and protocols of the Beyond Bilateral approach. But let's not forget the meat and potatoes of any good trauma therapy: mindfulness and self-compassion. These practices are the foundation upon which all the other work rests. Without them, we're just rearranging deck chairs on the Titanic, if you know what I mean.

So in this chapter, we're going to roll up our sleeves and get mindful. We'll explore how to use meditation to prepare the mind-body for deep healing, how to cultivate those all-important inner resources, and how to use self-compassion to kick negative beliefs and shame to the curb. Buckle up, buttercup - it's time to get our Zen on!

Meditation: Preparing the Mind-Body for Deep Healing

First things first: let's talk about meditation. Now, I know what some of you might be thinking. "Meditation? Isn't that just sitting around navel-gazing?" Well, yes and no. While meditation does involve a whole lot of sitting (or lying down, or walking - we're not picky), it's far from a passive activity. In fact, it's one of the most powerful tools we have for preparing the mind and body for deep, transformative healing.

So how does it work? At its core, meditation is simply the practice of bringing our attention to the present moment, over and over again. Whether we focus on the breath, a mantra, or the sensations in our body, the goal is to anchor ourselves in the here-and-now, rather than getting caught up in the endless chatter of our thoughts.

Sounds simple, right? Ha! As anyone who has ever tried to meditate can tell you, the mind has a funny way of wandering off to the far corners of the universe, usually right around the time we're trying to focus. But here's the thing: that's totally normal. The goal isn't to stop our thoughts (good luck with that!), but rather to notice when we've gotten hooked and gently bring ourselves back to the present.

So how does this relate to trauma therapy, you might ask? Well, let me count the ways:

1. **Regulating the Nervous System**: Trauma has a way of sending our nervous system into a tizzy - either revving us up into a state of hyperarousal or shutting us down into a state of hypoarousal. Meditation helps us find that sweet spot in the middle, the so-called "window of tolerance," where we can feel calm, grounded, and present.

2. **Enhancing Awareness**: Trauma can also wreak havoc on our ability to be present and aware. We might dissociate, numb out, or get lost in a spiral of negative thoughts. Meditation helps us cultivate a clearer, more focused awareness, so we can show up more fully for our own healing process.

3. **Building Resilience**: Let's face it - trauma therapy ain't for the faint of heart. It requires us to face some pretty gnarly stuff head-on. Meditation helps us build the inner strength and resilience we need to weather those storms. By practicing staying present with difficult

sensations and emotions, we learn that we can handle a whole lot more than we think.

So how do we actually do this thing? There are countless styles of meditation out there, from Zen to Vipassana to Transcendental Meditation. But for our purposes, a simple mindfulness practice will do just fine. Here's a basic recipe:

1. Find a quiet, comfortable spot where you won't be disturbed. (Pro-tip: put your phone on airplane mode. Trust me on this one.)

2. Sit or lie down in a way that feels stable and supported. You want to be relaxed, but not so comfy that you're likely to doze off.

3. Close your eyes (or leave them slightly open if that feels better) and take a few deep breaths. Notice the sensation of the breath moving in and out of your body.

4. Bring your attention to your chosen anchor - the breath, a mantra, or a body part (the belly or the feet work well). The goal isn't to clear your mind, but simply to notice when it wanders and gently bring it back.

5. When you get distracted (and you will!), just notice that it's happened and return your focus to your anchor. No judgment, no self-flagellation - just a simple, "Oops, there I go again," and a kind redirection of attention.

6. Start with just a few minutes and gradually build up to longer sessions. Even five minutes a day can make a big difference if practiced consistently.

Simple, right? Ha! Simple, yes. Easy, no. Meditation is a bit like going to the gym for your mind. It takes practice and patience. But the payoff is well worth it. By making meditation a regular part of your trauma therapy regimen, you're laying the groundwork for deeper, more sustainable healing.

Cultivating Inner Resources: Finding Your Center in the Storm

Alright, so we've got our meditation chops down. Now what? Well, one of the key skills we want to cultivate through our mindfulness practice is the ability to access our inner resources - those places of calm, groundedness, and stability that can anchor us in the midst of trauma's choppy waters.

You see, trauma has a way of making us feel like we're at the mercy of our emotions and memories. We might feel like we're being tossed around by the waves, with no solid ground to stand on. But the truth is, we all have inner resources we can draw on - even if they feel buried deep beneath the rubble of our trauma.

So what do these inner resources look like? They might be:

- A place in nature that feels peaceful and centering, like a quiet forest or a serene beach.

- A memory of a time when we felt safe, loved, and connected, like being held by a nurturing parent or spending time with a close friend.

- A felt sense of our own strength and resilience, like a time we overcame a challenge or stood up for ourselves.

- A spiritual connection to something greater than ourselves, whether that's God, the universe, or simply the web of life.

The key is to get to know these resources intimately, so we can call on them when we need them most. And that's where mindfulness comes in. By practicing turning our attention inward and really savoring these positive experiences, we start to wire them more deeply into our brains and bodies.

Here's a simple practice for cultivating your inner resources:

1. Start with a few minutes of meditation, just to settle your mind and body.

2. Bring to mind a resource that feels particularly resonant for you. It could be a place, a memory, a feeling, or an image.

3. Really flesh out the details of this resource. If it's a place, notice the sights, sounds, smells, and sensations. If it's a memory, put yourself back in that moment and relive it as vividly as you can. If it's a feeling, locate it in your body and breathe into it.

4. Spend a few minutes just marinating in this resource. Let it fill you up from head to toe.

5. When you're ready, take a deep breath and slowly open your eyes. Notice how you feel - chances are, you'll feel a bit more grounded, centered, and resourced.

The more you practice this, the more easily you'll be able to access your inner resources when you need them. And trust me, you're gonna need them. Because trauma therapy is a wild ride, and having a few go-to tools in your back pocket can make all the difference.

Self-Compassion: Giving Yourself the Love You Deserve

Alright, let's get real for a minute. Trauma sucks. It just does. And one of the suckiest parts of trauma is the way it can make us feel about ourselves. We might blame ourselves for what happened, feel ashamed of our symptoms, or just generally feel like a big ol' pile of garbage.

Enter self-compassion. Self-compassion is the radical act of treating ourselves with the same kindness, care, and understanding we would offer a good friend. It's about recognizing that we're all human, we all struggle, and we all deserve love and support - especially when we're going through something as tough as trauma.

Now, I know what you might be thinking. "But wait, isn't self-compassion just a fancy way of letting myself off the hook? Won't it make me weak and complacent?" Nope, nope, and nope. In fact, research shows that self-compassion is one of the most powerful predictors of resilience, motivation, and overall well-being. When we're kind to ourselves, we're more likely to bounce back from setbacks, take healthy risks, and pursue our goals with gusto.

So how do we cultivate self-compassion, especially in the face of trauma? Here are a few tips:

1. **Talk to Yourself Like a Friend**: When you notice yourself getting caught in a spiral of self-criticism or shame, ask yourself, "What would I say to a friend who was feeling this way?" Chances are, you'd be a whole lot nicer to them than you're being to yourself. Try extending that same kindness and understanding to yourself.

2. **Practice Mindfulness of Thoughts**: Our minds have a sneaky way of convincing us that our negative thoughts are the truth, the whole truth, and nothing but the truth. But thoughts are just thoughts - they're not facts. Practice noticing your self-critical thoughts with curiosity and distance, rather than getting hooked by them. You

might even try labeling them as "thinking" or "judging" to help create some space.

3. **Give Yourself a Break**: Trauma recovery is hard work. It's okay to take breaks, rest, and recharge. In fact, it's necessary. Make sure you're building in plenty of time for self-care, whether that's taking a bubble bath, going for a walk in nature, or just vegging out on the couch with a good book.

4. **Seek Out Support**: We're social creatures, wired for connection. When we're struggling, it's so important to reach out for support - whether that's to a therapist, a support group, or a trusted friend or family member. Knowing that we're not alone in our pain can be incredibly healing.

5. **Practice Self-Compassion Meditations**: There are tons of great self-compassion meditations out there that can help us cultivate a kinder, more loving relationship with ourselves. One of my favorites is the "Self-Compassion Break" by Kristin Neff. It goes like this:

- Take a few deep breaths and settle into your body.

- Bring to mind a situation that's causing you stress or pain.

- Notice any difficult emotions or sensations that arise.

- Place your hand on your heart (or wherever feels comforting) and say to yourself, "This is a moment of suffering. Suffering is a part of life. May I be kind to myself in this moment. May I give myself the compassion I need."

- Repeat these phrases a few times, really letting them sink in.

- Take a few more deep breaths and notice any shifts in your body or mind.

Simple, right? But don't underestimate the power of these small acts of self-kindness. When we practice treating ourselves with compassion, we start to rewire our brains for greater resilience, self-worth, and overall well-being.

Wrapping It Up

Whew, that was a lot of inner work! We covered some serious ground in this chapter - from meditation to inner resourcing to self-compassion. But here's the thing: these practices are the secret sauce of trauma therapy. They're what allow us to show up more fully, heal more deeply, and thrive more authentically.

Because at the end of the day, trauma recovery isn't just about fixing what's broken. It's about discovering our innate wholeness, wisdom, and strength. It's about learning to love and accept ourselves, even in the face of our most painful experiences. And it's about reconnecting with the beauty, joy, and resilience that have been within us all along.

So keep practicing, my friends. Keep breathing, keep resourcing, and keep giving yourself the compassion you so richly deserve. Because you are worth it. You are enough. And you are whole, even in the midst of your healing.

And always remember: if you get stuck, just come back to the breath. It's the simplest, most powerful tool we have for coming home to ourselves. One breath at a time, one moment at a time, we can do this. Together.

Happy mindful-ing, y'all!

Chapter 6 Resilience and Post-Traumatic Growth

Well, well, well. You've made it to the final chapter of this little trauma-healing soirée. Congratulations! You've faced your demons, ridden the EMDR roller coaster, and gotten up close and personal with your bodily sensations. You're practically a trauma-whispering ninja at this point.

But hold up - we're not quite done yet. Because as much as we'd all love to ride off into the sunset, trauma recovery in hand, the reality is a bit more complicated. Trauma has a sneaky way of popping back up when we least expect it, like a game of emotional whack-a-mole. Triggers, stressors, and good old-fashioned life challenges are bound to rear their ugly heads from time to time.

So how do we navigate this post-therapy world with grace, resilience, and a hefty dose of self-compassion? How do we not just survive, but thrive in the face of adversity? That's what we're going to explore in this final chapter. Buckle up, buttercup - it's time to get our post-traumatic growth on!

Building Resilience: Bouncing Back from Triggers and Stressors

First things first: let's talk about resilience. Resilience is the ability to bounce back from tough times, to adapt and recover in the face of adversity. It's the psychological equivalent of those inflatable punching bags that just keep popping back up, no matter how many times you knock them down.

Now, I know what you might be thinking. "But wait, I've been through some serious sh*t. How can I be resilient after all that?" And to that, I say: fair point. Trauma can take a serious toll on our resilience reserves. It can leave us feeling depleted, fragile, and like the smallest gust of wind could knock us over.

But here's the good news: resilience is a skill, not a fixed trait. It's something we can cultivate and strengthen over time, like a muscle. And just like with any muscle, it takes practice, patience, and a willingness to show up for ourselves, even when things get tough.

So how do we build our resilience muscles? Here are a few tips:

1. **Develop a Growth Mindset**: A growth mindset is the belief that our abilities and traits are malleable, not fixed. It's the idea that we can learn, grow, and improve with effort and practice. When we have a growth mindset, we're more likely to see challenges as opportunities for growth, rather than threats to our sense of self. We're more willing to take risks, learn from our mistakes, and keep pushing forward, even when things get tough.

2. **Cultivate a Support System**: We're social creatures, wired for connection. When we have a strong support system - whether that's friends, family, a therapist, or a support group - we're more likely to weather life's storms with resilience and grace. Reach out to your loved ones, let them know what you're going through, and lean on them when you need to. Remember: asking for help is a sign of strength, not weakness.

3. **Practice Self-Care**: Self-care isn't just bubble baths and face masks (although those are great too!). It's about taking care of ourselves on a deep, holistic level - physically, emotionally, mentally, and spiritually. It's about getting enough sleep, eating nourishing foods,

moving our bodies in ways that feel good, and making time for activities that bring us joy and relaxation. When we prioritize self-care, we're better equipped to handle whatever life throws our way.

4. **Develop a Toolkit of Coping Skills**: Remember all those fancy trauma therapy techniques you learned? The EMDR, the somatic work, the mindfulness meditations? Those are your coping skills toolkit. When a trigger or stressor pops up, you can reach into that toolkit and pull out a technique that works for you. Maybe it's a few minutes of deep breathing, or a quick body scan, or a self-compassion mantra. The more tools you have at your disposal, the more resilient you'll be in the face of adversity.

5. **Practice Gratitude**: Gratitude is the ultimate resilience booster. When we take time to appreciate the good things in our lives - no matter how small - we shift our focus from what's wrong to what's right. We cultivate a sense of abundance, rather than scarcity. And we remind ourselves that even in the darkest of times, there is still beauty and goodness to be found. Try keeping a gratitude journal, where you write down three things you're grateful for each day. Over time, you'll start to train your brain to scan for the positive, even in tough situations.

Now, I know what you might be thinking. "Easier said than done, Doc." And you're right. Building resilience takes time, effort, and a whole lot of self-compassion. There will be days when you feel like you're taking one step forward and two steps back. There will be moments when you want to throw in the towel and give up.

But here's the thing: resilience isn't about never getting knocked down. It's about getting back up, again and again. It's about facing our challenges with courage, vulnerability, and a willingness to learn and grow. And it's about remembering that we are so much stronger than we give ourselves credit for.

So keep practicing, my friends. Keep showing up for yourselves, even when it's hard. Keep reaching out for support, keep prioritizing self-care, and keep cultivating that unshakeable core of resilience that lives within you. Because you've got this. You really, truly do.

Envisioning and Manifesting Your Healed, Empowered Self

Alright, so we've got our resilience muscles flexed and ready to go. But what about the bigger picture? What does life look like beyond just coping with triggers and stressors? What does it mean to truly heal, to thrive, to step into our fullest, most empowered selves?

That's where the concept of post-traumatic growth comes in. Post-traumatic growth is the idea that we can actually emerge from our traumas stronger, wiser, and more resilient than before. It's the notion that our darkest struggles can be the very things that catalyze our greatest transformations, if we let them.

Now, I know what you might be thinking. "Post-traumatic growth? That sounds like a bunch of woo-woo nonsense." And I get it. When we're in the thick of trauma recovery, the idea of "growing" from our pain can feel like a cruel joke. But hear me out.

Post-traumatic growth isn't about sugarcoating our suffering or pretending that trauma is some kind of cosmic gift. It's not about bypassing our pain or rushing to forgiveness. It's about allowing ourselves to be changed by what we've been through, in ways that ultimately lead to greater wholeness, authenticity, and purpose.

So what does post-traumatic growth actually look like? It can manifest in many different ways, but here are a few common themes:

1. **Greater Self-Awareness**: Trauma has a way of shattering our assumptions about ourselves and the world around us. It can force us to confront parts of ourselves that we've long ignored or denied. And while this process can be painful, it can also lead to a deeper, more authentic sense of self. We may discover new strengths, values, and passions that we never knew we had. We may learn to set healthier boundaries, communicate our needs more clearly, and stand up for ourselves in ways we never could before.

2. **Deeper Relationships**: Trauma can also be a catalyst for more meaningful, authentic relationships. When we allow ourselves to be vulnerable with others, to share our stories and our struggles, we create space for real connection and intimacy. We may find that some relationships fall away, as we learn to let go of people who aren't aligned with our growth. But we may also discover new relationships that nourish and support us in profound ways.

3. **Renewed Sense of Purpose**: For many trauma survivors, the journey of healing can be a powerful catalyst for finding a new sense of purpose and meaning in life. We may feel called to use our experiences to help others, to raise awareness about trauma and mental health, or to create art and beauty from our pain. We may discover a

deeper sense of what truly matters to us, and start living our lives in greater alignment with those values.

4. **Increased Resilience**: As we navigate the ups and downs of trauma recovery, we naturally build our resilience muscles along the way. We learn that we can survive tough times, that we have the strength and the tools to cope with whatever life throws our way. We may even find that we're better equipped to handle future challenges, because we've already been through the fire and come out the other side.

5. **Greater Appreciation for Life**: Trauma has a way of putting things in perspective. When we've faced our own mortality, or the fragility of life, we may find ourselves savoring the small moments more fully. We may feel a deeper sense of gratitude for the people and experiences that bring us joy and meaning. We may even develop a kind of "tragic optimism," a belief that life is inherently meaningful, even in the face of great suffering.

So how do we cultivate post-traumatic growth? How do we allow ourselves to be transformed by our traumas, in ways that lead to greater wholeness and vitality? Here are a few practices to try:

1. **Envision Your Healed, Empowered Self**: Take some time to imagine your future self, the version of you that has moved through the pain of trauma and come out the other side. What does that self look like? How do they carry themselves, speak to themselves, show up in the world? What kind of life are they living, and how does it feel to inhabit that reality? The more vividly you can

imagine this healed, empowered self, the more you'll start to embody those qualities in the present moment.

2. **Practice Self-Reflection**: Post-traumatic growth requires a willingness to look within, to explore our thoughts, feelings, and beliefs with curiosity and compassion. Set aside some time each day for self-reflection, whether that's through journaling, meditation, or talking with a trusted friend or therapist. Ask yourself questions like: "What have I learned about myself through this experience? What values and priorities have become clearer to me? How do I want to grow and change as a result of what I've been through?"

3. **Seek Out New Experiences**: Growth often requires stepping outside of our comfort zones, trying new things, and embracing uncertainty. Look for opportunities to challenge yourself in healthy ways, whether that's taking a class, traveling somewhere new, or volunteering for a cause you care about. The more we expose ourselves to new perspectives and experiences, the more we open ourselves up to transformation.

4. **Find Meaning in Your Story**: One of the most powerful ways to cultivate post-traumatic growth is to find meaning and purpose in our struggles. This doesn't mean that our traumas happened "for a reason," or that we should be grateful for them. But it does mean that we can choose to use our experiences as fuel for positive change, both in our own lives and in the world around us. Look for ways to share your story, to connect with others who have been through similar struggles, and to use your voice for good.

5. **Celebrate Your Progress**: Post-traumatic growth is a journey, not a destination. It's important to celebrate your progress along the way, no matter how small or incremental it may feel. Take time to acknowledge your own strength, resilience, and courage. Give yourself credit for showing up, day after day, even when it's hard. And remember that healing is not a linear process - there will be ups and downs, setbacks and breakthroughs. But every step you take is a step towards greater wholeness and empowerment.

Maintaining Well-Being Beyond Therapy

Whew, we've covered a lot of ground in this chapter! We've explored resilience, post-traumatic growth, and the practices that can help us cultivate both. But before we wrap things up, I want to take a moment to talk about what comes next - how to maintain our well-being beyond the therapy room.

Because here's the thing: therapy is a powerful tool for healing and growth, but it's not a magic bullet. It's not a one-and-done deal. The work of trauma recovery is ongoing, and it requires a commitment to showing up for ourselves, day in and day out, long after we've said goodbye to our therapists.

So how do we do that? How do we maintain our hard-won progress, and continue to thrive in the face of life's challenges? Here are a few tips:

1. **Stay Connected to Your Support System**: Whether it's friends, family, a support group, or a spiritual community, it's so important to stay connected to the people who love and support us. Make time for regular check-ins, even if it's just a quick phone call or coffee date. And don't be afraid to reach out when you're

struggling - remember, asking for help is a sign of strength, not weakness.

2. **Keep Up with Your Self-Care Practices**: Those self-care practices that you learned in therapy? Keep doing them! Whether it's meditation, yoga, journaling, or taking a bubble bath, make sure you're prioritizing your own well-being on a daily basis. And if you find yourself slipping into old patterns of neglect or self-abandonment, gently redirect yourself back to those practices that nourish and sustain you.

3. **Stay Engaged with Your Passions and Purpose**: One of the most powerful ways to maintain our well-being is to stay connected to the things that bring us joy, meaning, and fulfillment. Whether it's a hobby, a creative pursuit, or a cause we care about, make sure you're carving out time for the things that light you up inside. And if you're still discovering what those things are, keep exploring! Try new things, take risks, and follow your curiosity.

4. **Keep Learning and Growing**: The journey of personal growth doesn't end when therapy does. There's always more to learn, more ways to stretch and evolve. Consider taking a class, reading a book, or attending a workshop on a topic that interests you. Surround yourself with people who inspire and challenge you to be your best self. And remember that growth is a lifelong process - there's no finish line, only the joy of the journey itself.

5. **Be Gentle with Yourself**: Finally, and perhaps most importantly, remember to be gentle with yourself. Trauma recovery is hard work, and there will be days when you feel like you're taking two steps forward and

one step back. There will be moments when old patterns and triggers resurface, and you'll wonder if you've made any progress at all. In those moments, take a deep breath, place a hand on your heart, and remind yourself that healing is not a linear process. It's a spiral, a dance, a journey of ups and downs. And every step you take, no matter how small or faltering, is a step in the right direction.

Conclusion

Well, my friends, we've reached the end of our little trauma-healing adventure. We've explored the ins and outs of EMDR, somatic work, and mindfulness. We've faced our demons, danced with our triggers, and learned to befriend our bodies and minds. We've discovered the power of resilience, the potential for post-traumatic growth, and the practices that can help us maintain our well-being for the long haul.

It's been a wild ride, hasn't it? But here's what I want you to remember, more than anything else: you are not your trauma. You are not defined by what happened to you, or by the symptoms and struggles that followed. You are a whole, worthy, and resilient being, with an unshakeable core of strength and wisdom that nothing can take away.

Yes, the road to healing is long and winding, and there will be plenty of bumps and detours along the way. But every step you take is a step towards greater freedom, wholeness, and vitality. Every moment of self-compassion, every flicker of hope, every glimmer of joy - these are the building blocks of a life well-lived, a life that is rich and full and meaningful, not in spite of your trauma, but because of it.

So keep going, my brave and beautiful friends. Keep showing up for yourselves, keep leaning on each other, and keep believing in the power of your own healing. Because you've got this. You really, truly do.

And remember: even on the darkest of days, when the shadows feel long and the path ahead feels uncertain, you are never, ever alone. You have an army of fellow survivors, healers, and helpers cheering you on, holding space for your pain, and believing in your inherent goodness. You have a universe that is conspiring in your favor, even when it doesn't feel like it. And you have a wise, loving, and unbreakable spirit within you, guiding you towards the light, one breath and one step at a time.

So here's to the journey, in all its messy, beautiful, and unexpected glory. Here's to the courage it takes to face our demons, and the grace it takes to love ourselves through the process. And here's to the life that awaits us on the other side - a life of resilience, growth, and unstoppable, unshakeable, unbreakable wholeness.

We've got this, my friends. Together, we've got this. And I, for one, can't wait to see what miracles unfold from here.

Conclusion

Well, folks, we've reached the end of the road. We've journeyed through the peaks and valleys of trauma recovery, with the trusty compass of the Beyond Bilateral approach guiding our way. We've faced our demons, befriended our bodies, and learned to love ourselves through the mess and the miracles of healing.

It's been a wild ride, hasn't it? But before we go our separate ways (and let's be real, after all this time together, I feel like we're practically family), let's take a moment to reflect on the insights and takeaways that will stick with us long after we close this book.

Key Insights and Takeaways

First and foremost, let's talk about the power of integration. The Beyond Bilateral approach is not just a fancy way of saying "throw everything at the wall and see what sticks." No, no, no. It's a carefully crafted framework that weaves together the best of EMDR, somatic therapy, and mindfulness practices, creating a synergistic effect that is greater than the sum of its parts.

By targeting trauma from multiple angles - the mental, the physical, and the spiritual - we're able to achieve a depth and breadth of healing that simply isn't possible with any one modality alone. It's like the difference between playing a simple melody on a single instrument versus a full symphony orchestra. The richness, the complexity, the sheer emotional impact - it's unparalleled.

But here's the thing: integration isn't just about the techniques and tools we use. It's about the way we show up as healers, as fellow humans walking this path of recovery. The Beyond Bilateral approach calls us to bring our whole selves to the work - our knowledge, our skills, our hearts, and our own hard-won wisdom. It invites us to meet our clients where they are, to honor their unique stories and strengths, and to hold space for the full spectrum of their experience - the pain and the joy, the despair and the hope, the darkness and the light.

In short, the Beyond Bilateral approach is not just a method - it's a way of being. A way of relating to ourselves, to each other, and to the world around us with greater compassion, curiosity, and wholeness.

And speaking of wholeness, let's talk about the ultimate goal of trauma recovery. It's not just about reducing symptoms or coping with triggers (although those are certainly important milestones along the way). No, the true aim of healing is to reclaim our birthright of wholeness - to remember and embody the truth of who we are beneath the layers of pain and protection.

You see, trauma has a way of shattering our sense of self, of fragmenting our identity into a thousand jagged pieces. We may feel like we're broken beyond repair, like we'll never be whole again. But the reality is, wholeness is our natural state. It's the ground of our being, the core of our essence. It's not something we need to strive for or earn - it's something we already are, something we simply need to uncover and claim.

The Beyond Bilateral approach is a powerful tool for this reclamation of wholeness. By integrating the mind, body, and spirit, we're able to access and express the fullness of our being. We're able to feel more alive, more connected, and more true to ourselves than ever before.

But here's the kicker: wholeness doesn't mean perfection. It doesn't mean we never feel pain or struggle or doubt. In fact, it means the opposite. Wholeness is about embracing the full spectrum of our humanity - the light and the dark, the beauty and the mess, the joy and the sorrow. It's about learning to love and accept ourselves, not in spite of our flaws and scars, but because of them.

As the great Leonard Cohen once said, "There is a crack in everything. That's how the light gets in." Our wounds, our imperfections, our struggles - these are not obstacles to wholeness, but gateways to a deeper, richer, and more authentic way of being. They are the cracks that let the light in, the openings that allow us to connect more fully with ourselves, with each other, and with the world around us.

So here's the invitation, my friends: embrace your cracks. Honor your scars. Love yourself fiercely, messily, and completely. Because that is the path to true aliveness, to genuine thriving, to unshakable wholeness.

An Inspiring Vision

And oh, what a vision that is! Can you imagine a world where we all walked in the fullness of our being? Where we showed up as our most authentic, radiant, and empowered selves? Where we met each other's pain with compassion, each other's joy with celebration, and each other's humanity with reverence?

That is the world I want to live in. That is the world I believe we're co-creating, one healing journey at a time. And that is the world that the Beyond Bilateral approach is pointing us towards, like a luminous North Star guiding us home.

But here's the thing: this vision isn't just about personal transformation. It's about collective transformation. It's about healing the wounds of our families, our communities, and our world. Because when we heal ourselves, we create ripples of change that extend far beyond our individual lives.

We become better partners, parents, and friends. We show up more fully in our work, our creativity, and our service. We inspire others to take the leap into their own healing journeys, creating a domino effect of growth and awakening.

And as more and more of us step into our wholeness, we start to shift the very fabric of our society. We create a culture of compassion, a culture of connection, a culture of courage. We challenge the systems and structures that perpetuate trauma and oppression, and we build new ones rooted in love, justice, and mutual thriving.

This is the vision that keeps me going, even on the hardest days. This is the vision that fuels my passion for this work, my commitment to walking alongside my clients as they navigate the twists and turns of recovery. Because I know that every moment of healing, every flicker of wholeness, every act of self-love and self-compassion - it all matters. It all contributes to the greater unfolding of our collective awakening.

And so, my dear friends, I invite you to hold this vision with me. To let it be the wind at your back, the fire in your belly, the light in your heart. To let it guide you forward, one brave and tender step at a time, into the life and the world that are waiting for you.

Because you matter. Your healing matters. Your wholeness matters. And together, we can create miracles beyond our wildest dreams.

A Final Word

And so, we come to the end of our journey (for now, at least - who knows what adventures await us on the other side of this book?). But before we go, I want to leave you with one final word of encouragement, one last rallying cry for the road ahead.

No matter where you are on your path of healing - whether you're just starting out or you've been at this for years, whether you feel like you're making progress or you're stuck in the muck, whether you're riding high on hope or you're drowning in despair - know this:

You are not alone. You are not broken. You are not a lost cause.

You are a brave and beautiful soul, a warrior of the heart, a navigator of the unknown. You are a miracle in motion, a force of nature, a revelation waiting to happen.

And even on the darkest of days, when the shadows feel long and the path ahead feels uncertain, remember this: you have everything you need within you to heal, to thrive, to rise. You have the strength, the resilience, the wisdom, and the grace. You have the love, the light, the laughter, and the magic.

You have the power to alchemize your pain into purpose, your wounds into wisdom, your scars into sacred art. You have the power to rewrite your story, to reclaim your sovereignty, to reshape your world.

And you have an army of fellow travelers cheering you on, every step of the way. You have the support of your ancestors, your guides, and your angels. You have the love of the universe itself, conspiring in your favor, always and forever.

So keep going, my beloved friend. Keep showing up, keep digging deep, keep leaning in. Keep daring to believe in your own brilliance, your own beauty, your own unbreakable wholeness.

Because the world needs your light, your love, your fierce and tender heart. The world needs your courage, your compassion, your unwavering commitment to healing and growth. The world needs you, in all your messy, magnificent, miraculous glory.

And I promise you this: every step you take, every crack you embrace, every moment of wholeness you claim - it all matters. It all makes a difference. It all leaves a legacy of love that will ripple out across space and time, healing hearts and transforming lives for generations to come.

So here's to the journey, my friend. Here's to the adventure of a lifetime. Here's to the wild and precious gift of your one, true, radiant self.

The world is waiting for you.

Let's go light it up.

Reference

1. Afifi, T.O., et al. (2014) 'Childhood maltreatment and substance use disorders among men and women in a nationally representative sample', Canadian Journal of Psychiatry, 59(11), pp. 606-613.

2. Bergmann, U. (2008) 'The neurobiology of EMDR: Exploring the thalamus and neural integration', Journal of EMDR Practice and Research, 2(4), pp. 300-314.

3. Bisson, J.I., et al. (2007) 'Psychological treatments for chronic post-traumatic stress disorder: Systematic review and meta-analysis', British Journal of Psychiatry, 190(2), pp. 97-104.

4. Bradley, R., et al. (2005) 'A multidimensional meta-analysis of psychotherapy for PTSD', American Journal of Psychiatry, 162(2), pp. 214-227.

5. Briere, J., and Scott, C. (2015) Principles of trauma therapy: A guide to symptoms, evaluation, and treatment. 2nd edn. Thousand Oaks, CA: Sage Publications.

6. Brown, S.H., et al. (2019) 'Somatic interventions for treating child and adolescent trauma', Journal of Child & Adolescent Trauma, 12(3), pp. 305-320.

7. Corrigan, F.M., and Hull, A.M. (2015) 'Neglect of the complex: Why psychotherapy for post-traumatic clinical presentations is often ineffective', BJPsych Bulletin, 39(2), pp. 86-89.

8. Courtois, C.A. (2008) 'Complex trauma, complex reactions: Assessment and treatment', Psychological Trauma: Theory, Research, Practice, and Policy, S(1), pp. 86-100.

9. Cozolino, L. (2017) The neuroscience of psychotherapy: Healing the social brain. 3rd edn. New York, NY: W.W. Norton & Company.

10. Felitti, V.J., et al. (1998) 'Relationship of childhood abuse and household dysfunction to many of the leading causes of death in adults: The Adverse Childhood Experiences (ACE) Study', American Journal of Preventive Medicine, 14(4), pp. 245-258.

11. Fisher, J. (2019) Sensorimotor psychotherapy in the treatment of trauma. New York, NY: Guilford Press.

12. Hase, M., et al. (2015) 'Eye movement desensitization and reprocessing (EMDR) therapy in the treatment of depression: A matched pairs study in an inpatient setting', Brain and Behavior, 5(6), e00342.

13. Herman, J.L. (2015) Trauma and recovery: The aftermath of violence - from domestic abuse to political terror. New York, NY: Basic Books.

14. Korn, D.L. (2009) 'EMDR and the treatment of complex PTSD: A review', Journal of EMDR Practice and Research, 3(4), pp. 264-278.

15. Leeds, A.M. (2016) A guide to the standard EMDR therapy protocols for clinicians, supervisors, and consultants. 2nd edn. New York, NY: Springer Publishing Company.

16. Levine, P.A. (2015) Trauma and memory: Brain and body in a search for the living past. Berkeley, CA: North Atlantic Books.

17. Ogden, P., and Fisher, J. (2015) Sensorimotor psychotherapy: Interventions for trauma and attachment. New York, NY: W.W. Norton & Company.

18. Porges, S.W. (2011) The polyvagal theory: Neurophysiological foundations of emotions, attachment, communication, and self-regulation. New York, NY: W.W. Norton & Company.

19. Schore, A.N. (2012) The science of the art of psychotherapy. New York, NY: W.W. Norton & Company.

20. Shapiro, F. (2018) Eye movement desensitization and reprocessing (EMDR) therapy: Basic principles, protocols, and procedures. 3rd edn. New York, NY: Guilford Press.

21. Siegel, D.J. (2012) The developing mind: How relationships and the brain interact to shape who we are. 2nd edn. New York, NY: Guilford Press.

22. Solomon, R.M., and Shapiro, F. (2008) 'EMDR and the adaptive information processing model: Potential mechanisms of change', Journal of EMDR Practice and Research, 2(4), pp. 315-325.

23. Steinberg, M., and Schnall, M. (2001) The stranger in the mirror: Dissociation - the hidden epidemic. New York, NY: HarperCollins.

24. van der Kolk, B.A. (2014) The body keeps the score: Brain, mind, and body in the healing of trauma. New York, NY: Viking.

25. van der Kolk, B.A., et al. (2007) 'A randomized clinical trial of eye movement desensitization and reprocessing (EMDR), fluoxetine, and pill placebo in the treatment of posttraumatic stress disorder: Treatment effects and long-term maintenance', Journal of Clinical Psychiatry, 68(1), pp. 37-46.

26. Wampold, B.E., et al. (2010) 'What works in the treatment of PTSD? A meta-analytic review of randomized clinical trials', Clinical Psychology Review, 30(8), pp. 923-933.

27. Wesselmann, D., et al. (2012) 'EMDR as a treatment for improving attachment status in adults and children', Revue Européenne de Psychologie Appliquée/European Review of Applied Psychology, 62(4), pp. 223-230.

28. WHO (2013) Guidelines for the management of conditions specifically related to stress. Geneva: World Health Organization.

29. Wilkinson, M. (2019) Changing minds in therapy: Emotion, attachment, trauma, and neurobiology. New York, NY: W.W. Norton & Company.